IMMERSION

A Pocket Guide to Sea Bathing and Winter
Swimming

Jérôme CLOCHARD

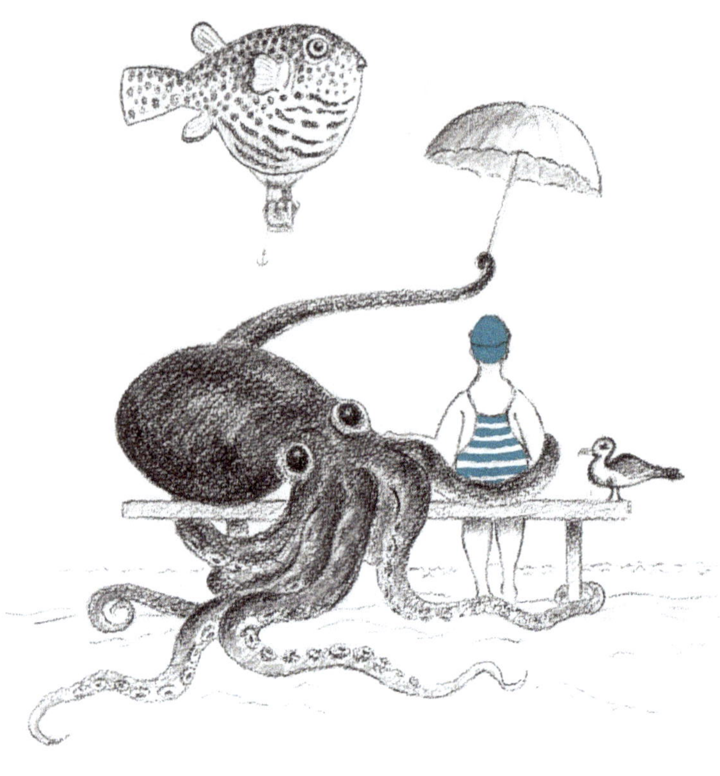

"Free man, you will always cherish the sea"

Introduction

This little guide to sea bathing shares insights gained through encounters, readings, personal experiences, and a profound connection with the sea. It extends an invitation to joyfully embrace sea bathing or swimming, demystifying the practice, unveiling its countless virtues, and explaining in simple terms the physiological mechanisms behind it.

Sea bathing is a communion with nature, embodying a philosophy, and ultimately a lifestyle that blends the aquatic with the marine. It stands as the ultimate ticket to physical health, mental well-being, and overall wellness.

As a child, I had the privilege of living on the island of Houat in Brittany for five years, a period that initiated my passionate relationship with the ocean. After several years of dedicated sailing in the Gulf of Morbihan, I worked as a diver and combat swimmer in the military for over a decade—an extraordinary experience of immersion and connection with the ocean.

Enthusiastic about open sea swimming, I later started a small, friendly winter swimming group on the Fouras peninsula in Charente-Maritime: the Pelagos Swimming Social Club.

Today, the turquoise waters of Finistère's wild beaches welcome me daily as I practice sea bathing with ever-renewed joy.

I would like to express my heartfelt gratitude to Jaimie

Monahan, an extreme swimmer from New York and multiple international record holder, who contributed to this book with immense kindness and humility. The character featured in this guide is inspired by her.

My deepest thanks also go to Dr. Guillaume Barucq, an author and passionate expert on the benefits of seawater, as well as a surfer and swimmer, who read, corrected, and validated the texts in this guide.

Jérôme Clochard

Table of contents

Preface by Jaimie Monahan

Jaimie Monahan is a three-time Guinness World Record Holder in ice, winter, and ultramarathon swimming. Jaimie is from New York City and has enjoyed open water swimming and set records on all seven continents from Antarctica to the Arctic. She has completed non-stop solo swims up to 45 hours and 183 km in duration, including some of the longest and coldest recorded swims in history. Jaimie is the Queen of Manhattan Island with 32 completions of this iconic swim

Every few years, popular science seems to come up with a new list of things that are good and bad for our health. Recently, open water swimming, in particular cold water immersion, has been touted as a cure-all for many aspects of physical and mental wellness.
But unlike many other remedies that may fade in and out of style, open water swimming is truly one of the best things you can do to stay happy and healthy. As a lifelong swimmer, the water has given me fitness, friendships, fun and adventure. There are so many benefits. Swimming is probably the only skill that can save your life, but also feels amazing.
Swimmers are hedonists. In the water we feel refreshed, supported, free from gravity. Cold water in particular gives a feeling of exhilaration and well being. And while you can swim alone, braving the elements with a group forms deep social connections. Swimmers around the world have an immediate shared experience that is a strong and unique bond.

Other life changing aquatic connections are with nature. I've been fortunate to encounter turtles, penguins, fish, and seals during my swims on all seven continents.

And while the most impressive structures to see while swimming around my home island of Manhattan are man-made skyscrapers, I've also been able to commune with glaciers and icebergs on my swims in remote places, some rarely seen by humans.

Whether we bathe or swim in lakes, rivers and the sea, we become part of nature. In some ways every swim is an eco-swim because there is no way to love the water without becoming a conservationist and a water ambassador.

Jérôme Clochard is an amazing artist, writer, craftsman, and swimmer. I adore his charming il-lustrations and helpful words and hope you do too.

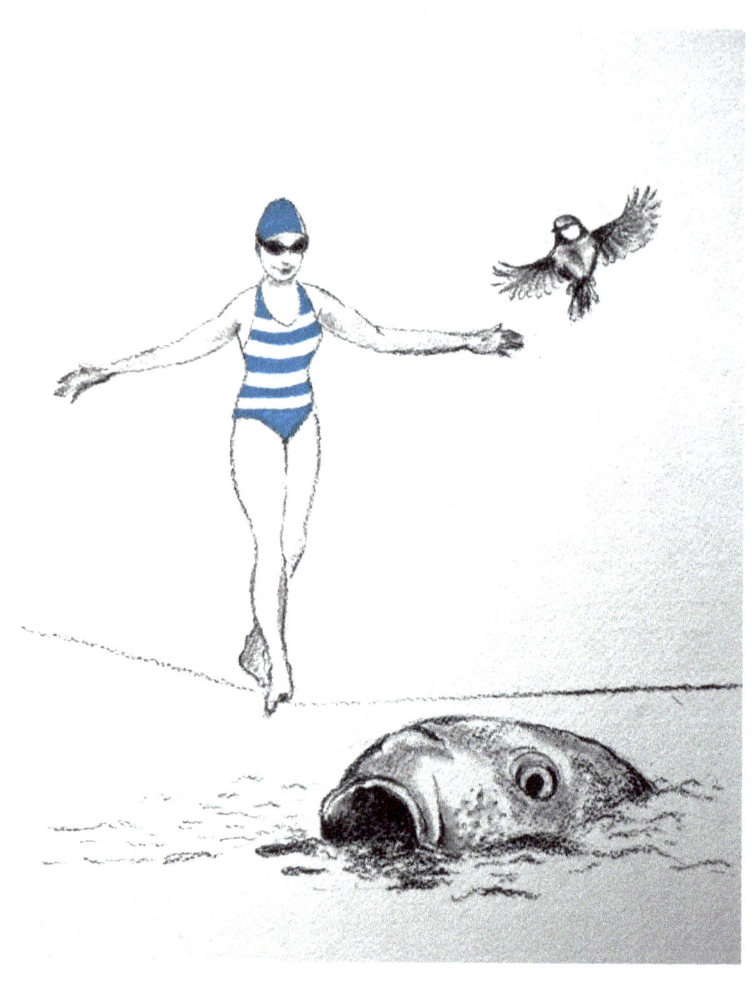

1. Water Through the Ages

For millennia, water in general and the sea in particular have been used to treat physical, psychological, and spiritual ailments.

Water contains healing; it is the simplest, cheapest, and—if used correctly—the safest remedy...
Sébastien Kneipp

Archaeological discoveries suggest that the use of hot springs dates back approximately 20,000 years.

By the 10th century BC, the Greeks had already established a well-documented practice of cold bathing, as attested by historians.

By the 4th century BC, the renowned physician Hippocrates recognized the benefits of bathing and began prescribing it as a treatment. The Egyptians also continued this practice in specialized establishments.

At the heart of Roman baths, hot and cold immersions became both a health necessity and a luxury, defining the culture of this civilization.

In the 2nd century, Claudius Galen, a prominent researcher and physician to gladiators and several Roman emperors, advocated for and meticulously described the stages of bathing: the changing room, the warm chamber, the very hot bath, and finally, the cold water pool.

Since antiquity, Japan has practiced a custom known as misogi—the purification of mind and body through water. This ritual involves immersing oneself in the icy waters of a waterfall or the sea.

Vikings developed a strong tradition of cold-water bathing, which has been passed down through generations in Scandinavian regions, and remains an integral part of their culture today.

The Middle Ages in Europe, however, marked a significant shift: there was a widespread aversion to and fear of the sea (Leroy, freely translated from French), and personal hygiene practices were largely abandoned.

In the 16th century, Ambroise Paré revived interest in the beneficial properties of seawater.

The 17th century saw the rise of sixty bathing establishments in England, thanks to Dr. Floyer's therapeutic experiments with water.

Dr. Richard Russel penned the first modern treatise on the healing benefits of seawater, titled The Use of Sea Water, in 1753. That same year, he founded the renowned Brighton Bathing Institute.

In the 1850s in Germany, Father Sébastian Kneipp became deeply interested in the therapeutic virtues of water, particularly cold water, and successfully cured his own tuberculosis—a disease considered incurable at the time. He popularized hydrotherapy by drawing on the work of Dr. Hahn and his own experiences. Kneipp wrote a book on the subject titled My Water-Cure and became known as the Water Doctor.

In France, 1847 marked the establishment of the first seawater therapy center in Sète by Mademoiselle Hirsch, followed by the opening of the first marine hospital in Berck-sur-Mer in 1861.

The term thalassotherapy was coined in 1865 by Dr. La Bonnardière, encompassing treatments using seawater, algae, sand and the marine climate.

Around 1950, Dr. Salmanoff, who had been Lenin's personal physician, pioneered capillotherapy through hot baths. This technique aimed to stimulate the microvessels of blood and lymph, which are crucial to our health. He detailed this approach in his book Les mille chemins de la guérison (The Thousand Paths to Healing).

Throughout the 20th century, thalassotherapy continued to evolve, taking on a more therapeutic focus.

Since the 1990s, the world of sports has shown great interest in the effects of cold baths on physical recovery and pain management.

From 2015 onwards, sea bathing—particularly winter swimming—has made a comeback in health and wellness circles. Its numerous benefits are being rediscovered.

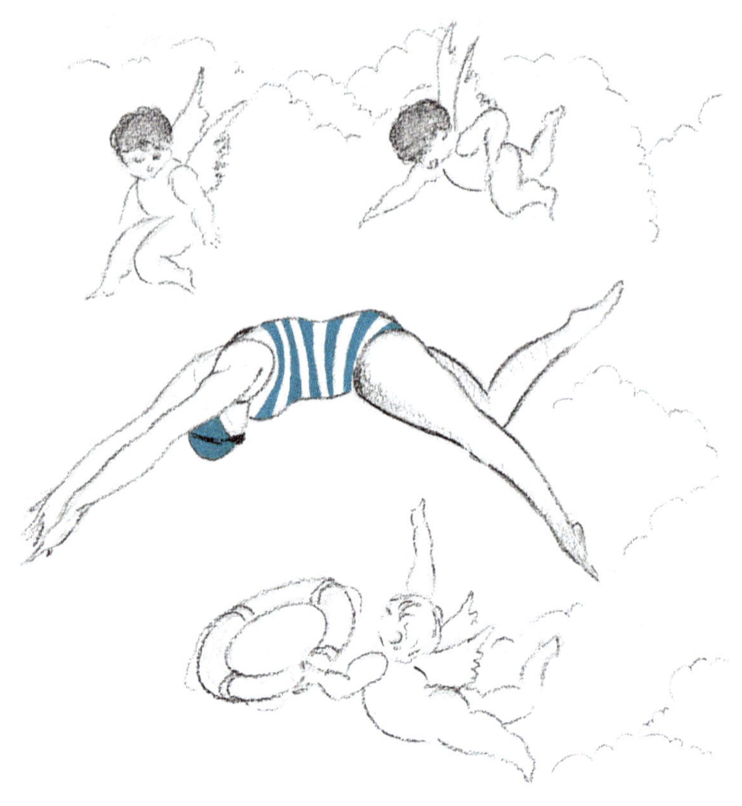

2. Sea Bathing,
a communion with Nature

Sea bathing is a communion with nature and a rendezvous with oneself: a sensory experience that embodies humility, mindfulness, trust, joy, and freedom.

The act of sea bathing quite literally pulls us out of our daily routines and immerses us in the heart of nature, with its rhythms, seasons, rules, and energy...

We receive and learn from the sea: the wind, the weather, the waves, the currents, the tides, the temperature, and the local flora and fauna.
Nature calls the shots, and we adapt. Let's approach it with respect and a curiosity to better understand it.

Through this connection, we gain a deeper sense of self-awareness: discovering our true nature, our sensitivities, the resilience of our bodies, their adaptability, and their limitations.

Let's set aside our preconceptions.

Let's ignite all of our senses, embrace the briny scents of the sea, the gentle caress of the water as it supports and glides over our body, the currents, the waves, the subtle changes in temperature.

Let's take in the ever-changing scenery, the colors of the sea and sky, the clouds drifting overhead; listen to the waves lapping at the shore and the breeze whistling past our wet skin.

Let's be fully present in this moment—we are in the heart of nature.

Naturally, swimming in the sea can also be a delightful and social activity with friends, offering rich interactions and plenty of joyful moments.

Let's respect this environment of which we are a part.

Each dip brings us complete serenity!

(NB Before heading to the beach, take a moment to review chapter 16: How to enjoy Sea Bathing: Some Advice).

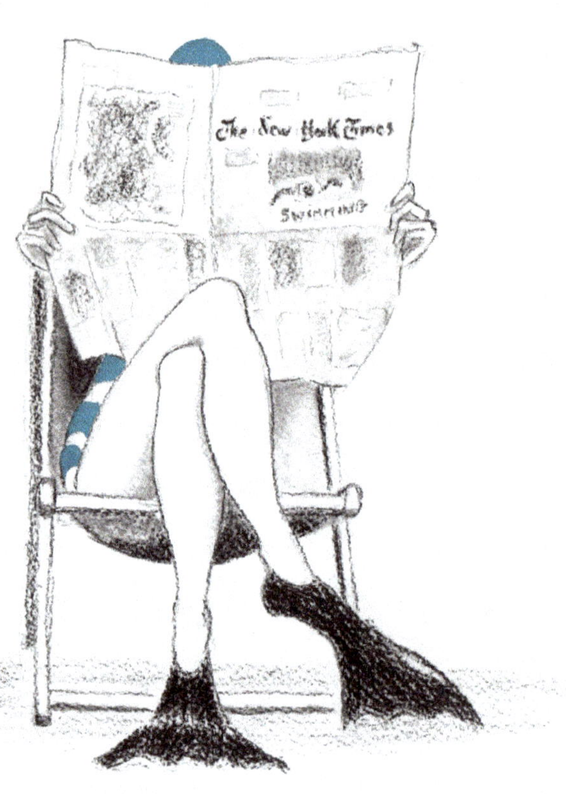

The New York Times
Swimming

3. Sea Bathing, a deeply Relaxing and holistic experience

Immersing ourselves in the sea offers an immediate and powerful relaxation effect, washing away negative thoughts, opening our mind, and freeing our body as we float weightlessly. This experience brings a profound sense of fulfillment.

The marine environment captures our attention and focus, directing our thoughts to our sensations. All our senses become alert and receptive.
In this state, we don't produce negative, stressful, or anxiety-inducing thoughts, we're simply receptive to the experience!

Unconsciously, we reconnect with an ancient and comforting sensation—that of a fetus floating in amniotic fluid.

Dr. Guillaume Barucq notes that sea bathing has a significant impact on the nervous system, offering both antidepressant and anti-anxiety effects.

The all-encompassing massage provided by the living waters promotes muscle and mental relaxation and proves particularly rejuvenating.
The sound of waves, the sulfur-rich air, and the weightlessness of our bodies in water are all incredibly soothing.

The decomposition of phytoplankton and algae releases bromine and the well-known sulfur compounds, which are more prevalent in the Atlantic and at higher latitudes. These elements are incredibly effective in combating fatigue and stress, making them conducive to relaxation.
They're responsible for the distinctive "iodine-like" scent we associate with the sea.

We emerge from each swim feeling calm and peaceful !

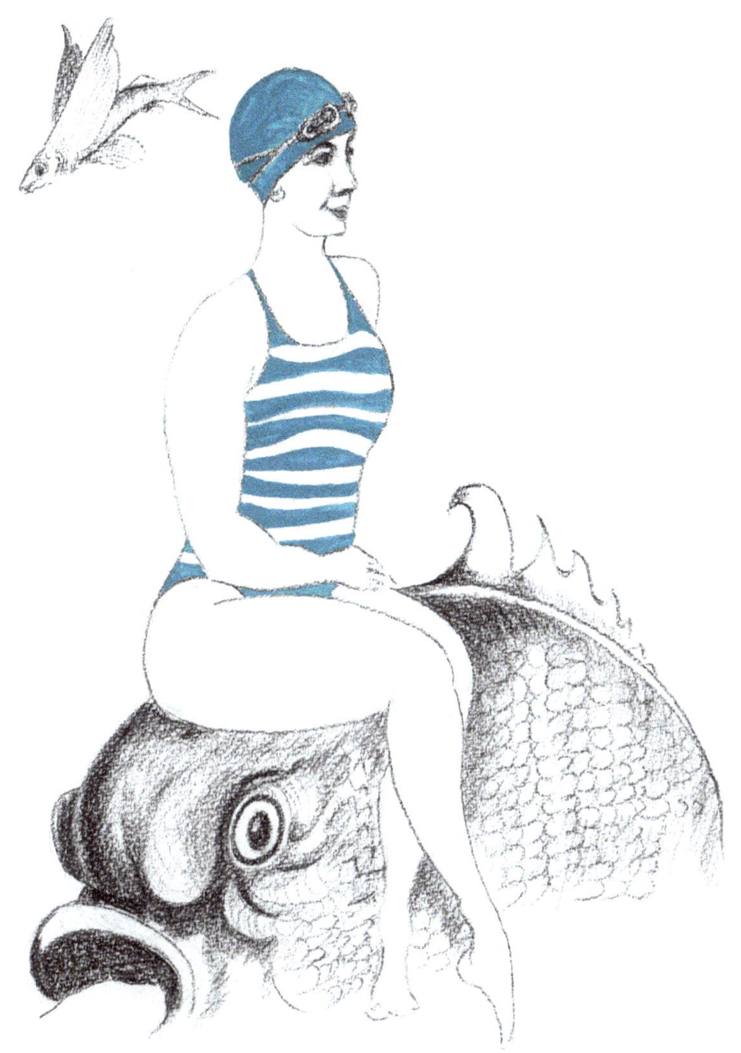

4. Invigorating, sea bathing boosts our energy and confidence

Regular swimmers often surprise others with their health, vitality, and daily enthusiasm.

Sea bathing has a genuinely positive effect on the psyche, often described as a feeling of euphoria. We always feel a sense of satisfaction after a swim, a sort of guarantee of joy and good spirits, regardless of the circumstances.

We've pushed past prejudices, shaken off our laziness, and braved unfavorable weather and frigid waters to immerse ourselves or swim. Sometimes, we've even managed to drag a friend along with us all these little triumphs make our day.

There's a real sense of renewal that washes over us, a feeling of accomplishment and pride in what we've done. Once completely warmed up, we experience general well-being, inner calm, renewed energy, and a brightened mood.

Regular sea bathing enhances our relationships with others, boosting our self-esteem and confidence.

Often, to fit this ritual into our schedule or to avoid the crowds, we head to our favorite beach in the early morning. The sea waits patiently for us there. As dawn breaks, nature reveals itself in all its beauty—

the sea, a canvas of blue-green hues, the air filled with briny scents. It's a welcoming embrace, and we relish this magical display, a unique and profound communion of the elements.

After every swim in the sea, we feel a deep sense of gratitude towards nature for all it gives us!

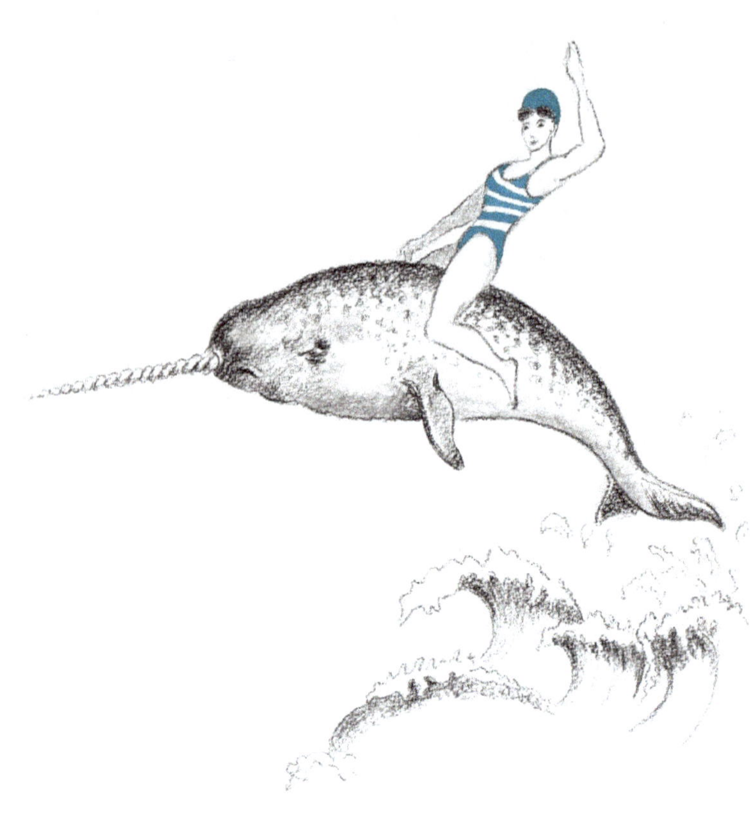

5. Replenishing With Minerals and Trace Elements

The sea is the original life-giving fluid, the birthplace of all living things. Biologist and physiologist René Quinton explains that we carry a living aquarium within us, highlighting the stark similarity between seawater and our blood plasma, particularly in their identical proportions of mineral salts.

This resemblance allows our bodies to readily absorb the essential minerals crucial for our functioning—magnesium, calcium, sodium, potassium, and others—along with trace elements like iodine, selenium, silicon, zinc, chromium, and manganese. These nutrients are absorbed through our skin and respiratory system during sea bathing, sometimes through involuntary absorption!

After fifteen minutes in the water, our bodies soak up these precious resources, distributing them throughout our system via capillaries and plasma, delivering them wherever they're needed.

Some of these elements are rare in our diets or difficult for our bodies to absorb from food alone.

For example, sea bathing is especially recommended for adequate iodine levels, which is essential for our bodies. This trace element plays significant roles in thyroid hormone function, cell maturation, body temperature regulation, energy expenditure, and protein synthesis.

The magnesium, sodium, and potassium in seawater greatly benefit muscle function, while the calcium is good for our bones.

The sea is truly a treasure trove, a cornucopia of health benefits. Regular sea bathing is like a rejuvenating tonic for our bodies.

(NB For optimal absorption, apply organic sunscreen after the bath, and wait an hour after leaving the water before rinsing off.)

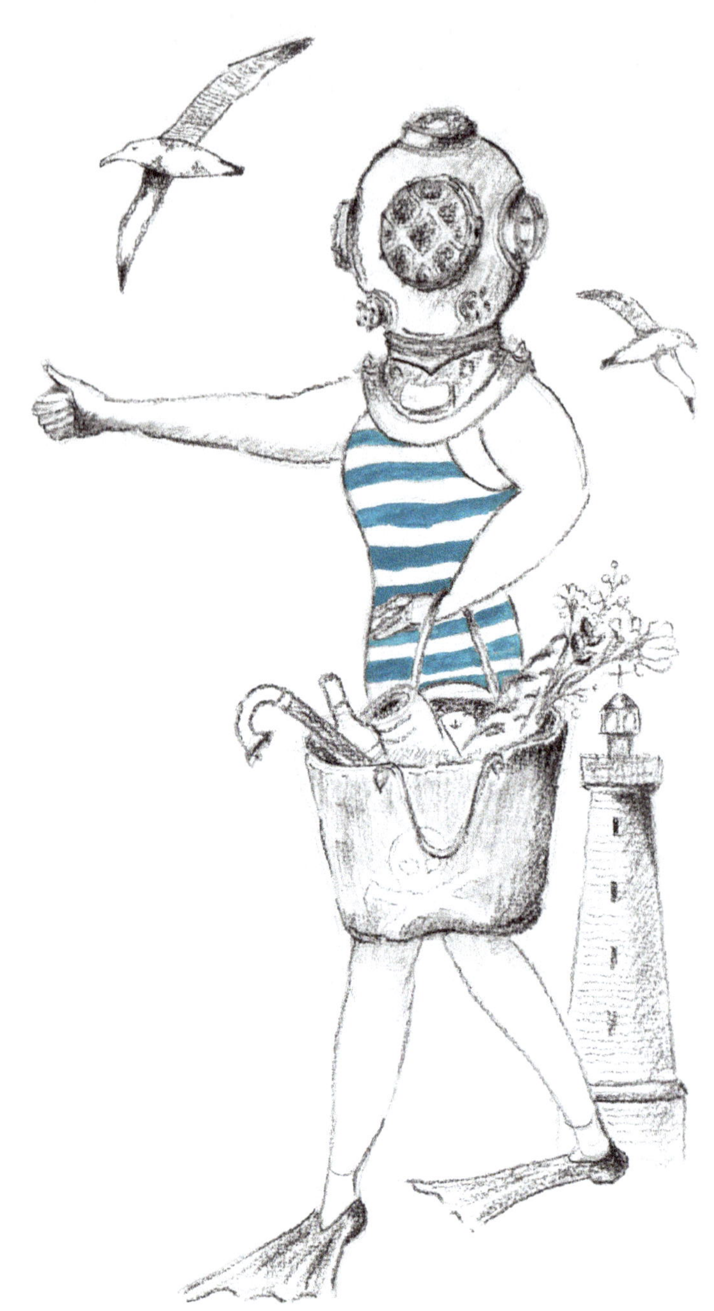

6. The Positive Impact of the Sea's Negative Ions

The higher the concentration of negative ions in a space, the greater its positive health effects. The surf, waves, and waterfalls, through their constant movement, break the structure of water molecules, releasing numerous electrons and creating a high concentration of charged atoms. These atoms, having captured new electrons, are known as negative ions.

Negative ions reach us primarily through respiration and promote both oxygen penetration in the lungs and exchanges between cells. This improves our physical capabilities—metabolism, strength, reflexes, endurance, recovery, sleep, mood, immunity—and mental faculties.

These negative ions have the ability to clean the air by removing dust, bacteria, germs, and pollutants. They also neutralize the more harmful positive ions that cause stress, fatigue, headaches, and general discomfort.

Negative ions have a favorable influence on overall lung function and help combat respiratory diseases, particularly asthma.

When the sea doesn't call us for a swim, walking alongside it can also provide us with numerous benefit.

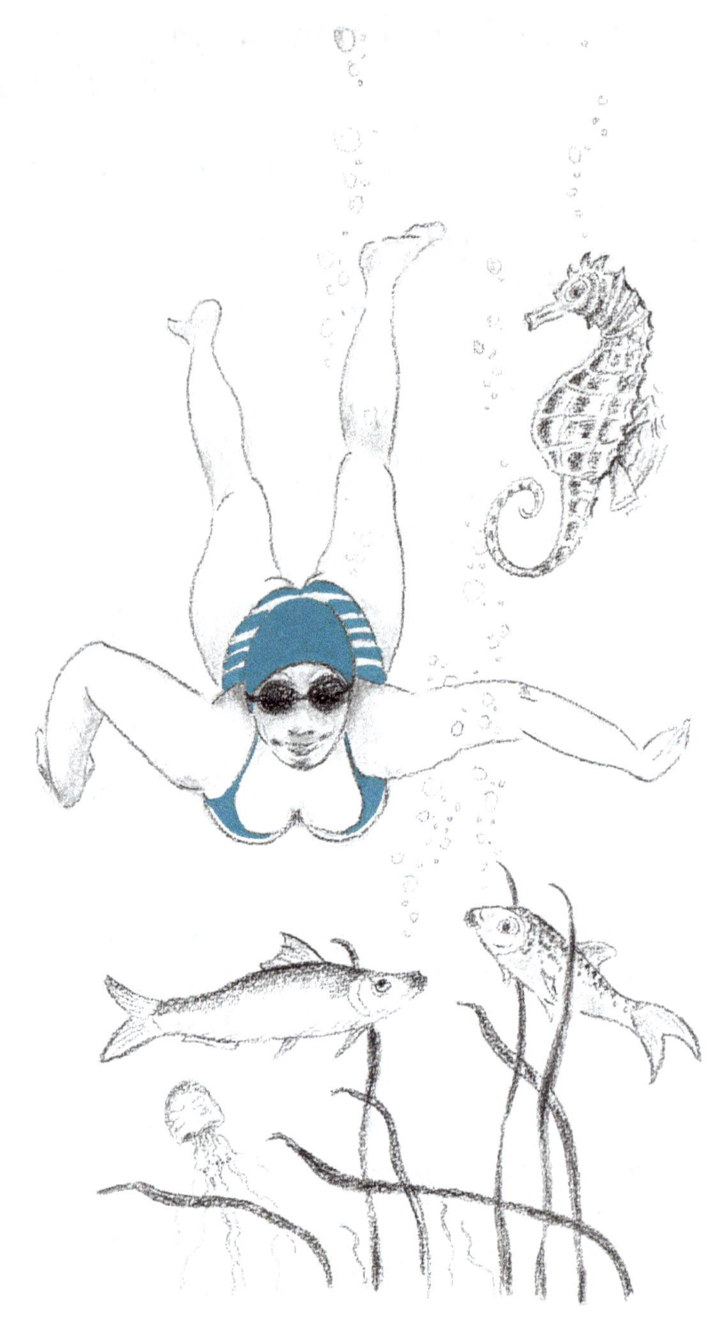

7. Easing Joint Pains

Thanks to buoyancy, our body weight is reduced to about a tenth in seawater. This state of near-weightless allows us to move our joints freely and fully, without significant muscle strain or risk of injury.

Sea bathing is especially beneficial for older adults. The water allows for gentle movement without impact or strain, particularly on vulnerable joints.

Swimming in the sea provides a thorough, full-body workout that tones muscles evenly and gently. It also improves motor coordination and boosts lung capacity.

Regular weekly sea bathing often helps reduce back pain, arthritis discomfort, and rheumatic aches.
Moreover, the natural composition of seawater has a soothing, pain-relieving effect. These benefits can be further enhanced by the body's release of endorphins when swimming in cool or cold water.

The backstroke is considered the ideal swimming style.

Breaststroke with the head underwater is also recommended, especially in the sea, as it doesn't put too much strain on the lower back and neck. Freestyle, while more technically demanding, is another excellent choice. It requires good breathing coordination and flexibility in the cervical vertebrae.

Whether you're swimming or simply moving about, go at your own pace. Focus on wide, slow movements, don't overexert yourself, and listen to your body.

No records need to be broken to reap multiple benefits.

Each dip in the sea liberates us!

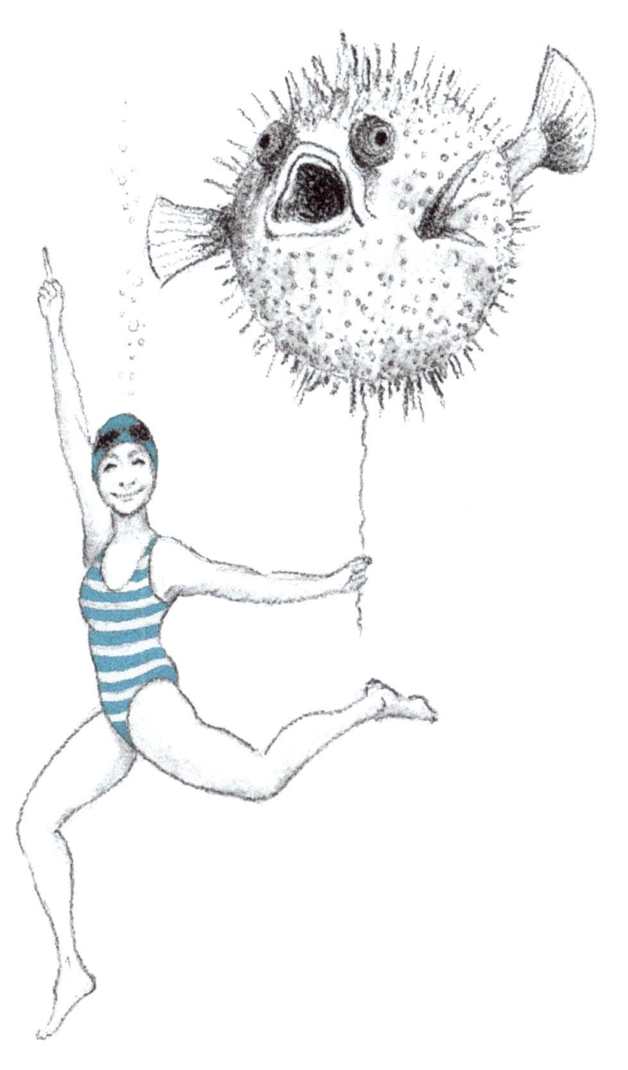

8. Sea Bathing Benefits Our Blood Circulation, Supports Cardiovascular Function, and Promotes Healthy Lymphatic Drainage

Temperature variations directly affect our capillaries, causing them to either dilate or contract—a phenomenon known as vasomotricity. This stimulation significantly enhances the health of our blood vessels.

Engaging in swimming or other dynamic activities while in the sea provides all the cardiovascular benefits of any sport: it lowers heart rate, improves blood pressure, and helps maintain or even build muscle.

Seawater, wherever we are, is always cooler than body temperature. Immersion immediately causes a contraction of superficial capillary vessels across the entire body and increased circulation to internal organs at higher pressure.

As we leave the water, these vessels dilate again (vasodilation), restoring peripheral circulation.

This invigorating workout for our vascular system—veins and arteries—is highly beneficial for combating venous insufficiency, relieving heavy legs, and improving our overall health.

This process benefits our blood pressure, heart function, and entire body.

An adult's circulatory system comprises roughly 100,000 kilometers of veins and arteries, with over 80% being micro-capillaries—tiny, hair-thin vessels. The brain alone contains 100 kilometers of these micro-capillaries.
These micro-vessels play a crucial role in delivering oxygen and nutrients to our cells.

By age 50, it's estimated that without proper stimulation, half of these tiny vessels may no longer function effectively, leading to gradual degeneration.
It is therefore essential to maintain this network.

Moving and swimming in seawater also stimulates lymphatic circulation through motion and massage, aiding in toxin drainage.

Lymph, which amounts to 6-10 liters circulating in our body, acts as our internal cleansing system—removing fat, bacteria, viruses, and microbes—in conjunction with our bloodstream. Since it lacks a pump like the heart, it's important to invigorate and facilitate its circulation to keep it flowing smoothly and efficiently.

The sea provides deep irrigation for our bodies!

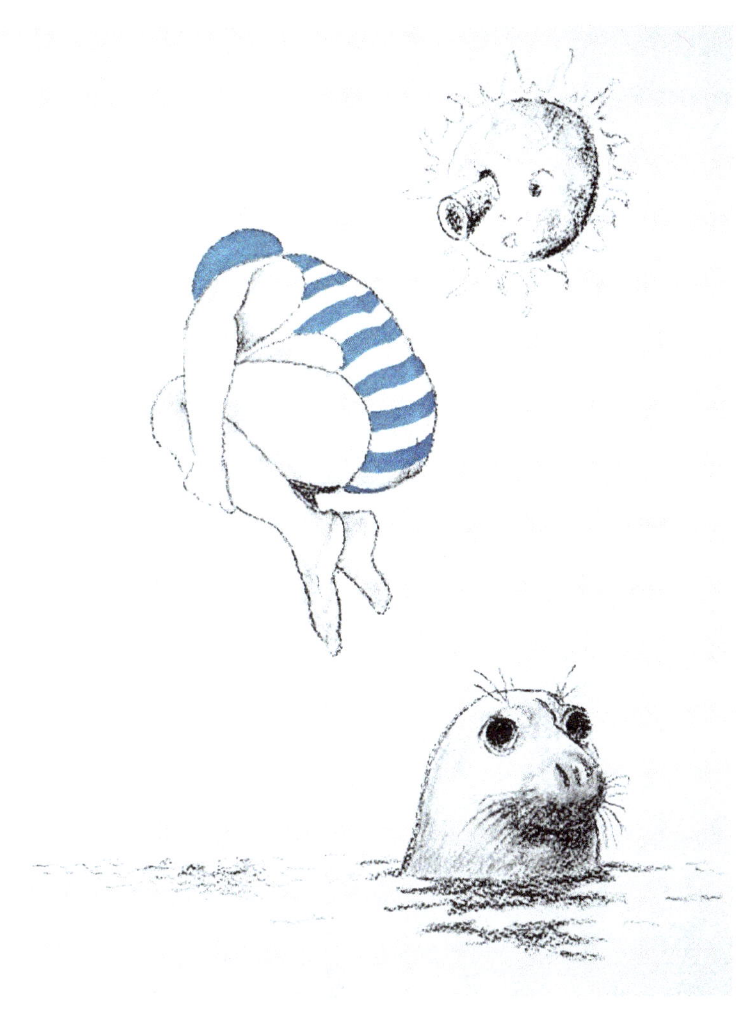

9. Strengthening Our Immune System

The sea contains certain trace elements that our bodies absorb while bathing. These elements turn out to be an excellent booster for our immune system.

Professor José Miguel Sempere, a medical researcher in immunology, suggests through numerous experiments that seawater—thanks to its minerals and trace elements—helps cells maintain their immune capacity and longevity, and may even stimulate their development.

Bathing, swimming, and breathing oxygen-rich sea air help to clear and cleanse our nasal passages and respiratory tracts, effectively eliminating microbes, allergens, and pathogens.

Dr. Guillaume Barucq conducted a study on regular sea bathers—those who take at least one weekly dip throughout the year in swimwear—with an average age of 57. These individuals rarely fall ill: 71% never catch a cold, their previous nose and ear infections cease, and 70% do not take any medication.

Moreover, they exhibit a much higher libido than average!

Sea bathing is our ticket to good health!

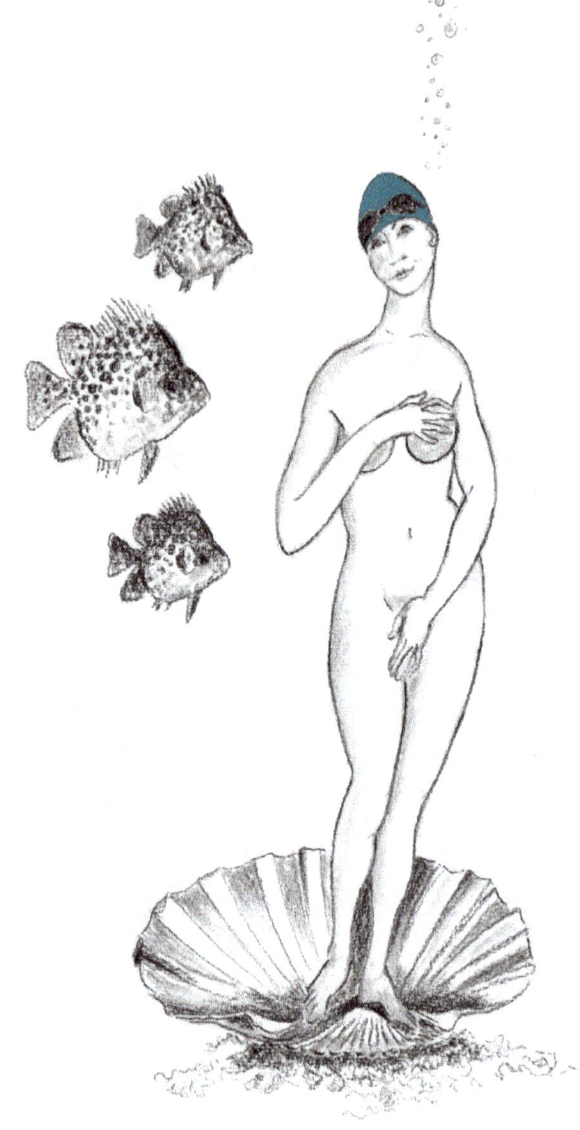

10. Excellent for Weight Regulation

Regular sea baths naturally help regulate body mass index, making them invaluable allies in weight management.

Swimming, movement, or exercises performed while bathing result in caloric expenditure due to the muscular effort involved. In fact, swimming is one of the most effective activities for burning calories.

Thirty minutes of butterfly stroke burns an average of 380 calories.
Thirty minutes of breaststroke burns 340 calories.
Thirty minutes of freestyle or backstroke burns 250 calories.

To keep things interesting and effective, don't shy away from mixing up your strokes, movements, and intensity levels.

On top of the calories burned through exercise, there's also the energy expended through thermoregulation. This natural mechanism works to maintain our body temperature at 37°C (98.6°F), especially in vital organs.

Since water conducts cold 25 times more effectively than air, the body works hard to maintain its internal temperature when immersed in the sea.

This remarkable ability of our body leads to a significant energy expenditure, burning even more calories as the water temperature drops.

An hour of leisurely swimming in a heated pool at 26°C (79°F) burns about 500 calories.
The same hour-long swim in a chilly 13°C (55°F) sea would burn 41% more calories!

Moreover, after a cold-water swim, our body continues to warm up well after we've left the water, depending on how long we were in.

Cold water consumes more energy than exercise!

Feel free to treat yourself to a pastry from your favorite bakery every now and then!
For your information, one butter croissant = a smile + a treat + a shared moment… And incidentally, 210 calories!

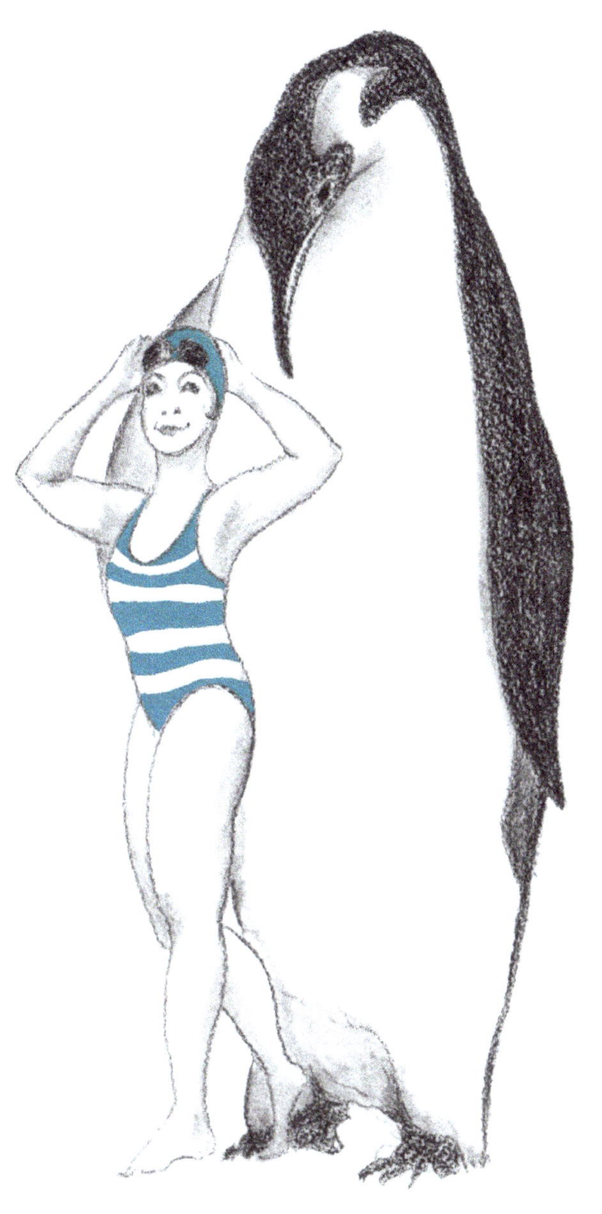

11. Toning the Skin

Contact with fresh seawater has a toning and anti-aging effect on the skin and face.

Thanks to its composition and rich array of minerals and trace elements, seawater provides hydration and radiance. It helps balance, maintain, and regenerate our skin cells, thereby slowing down the aging process.

The sea's antiseptic and anti-inflammatory properties soothe and improve various skin conditions such as herpes, eczema, hives, acne, and psoriasis.
(NB Caution: no bathing with an open wound!)

The presence of salt also acts as a gentle exfoliant, naturally removing dead skin cells with each bath, leaving our skin smoother and softer.

Cool water baths have the added benefit of firming the skin: vasoconstriction stimulates superficial microcirculation, improving skin appearance and suppleness.

The cosmetics industry is increasingly turning to marine resources in the formulation of its skincare and wellness products.
These ingredients possess unique chemical and biological properties not found on land, making them highly valuable.

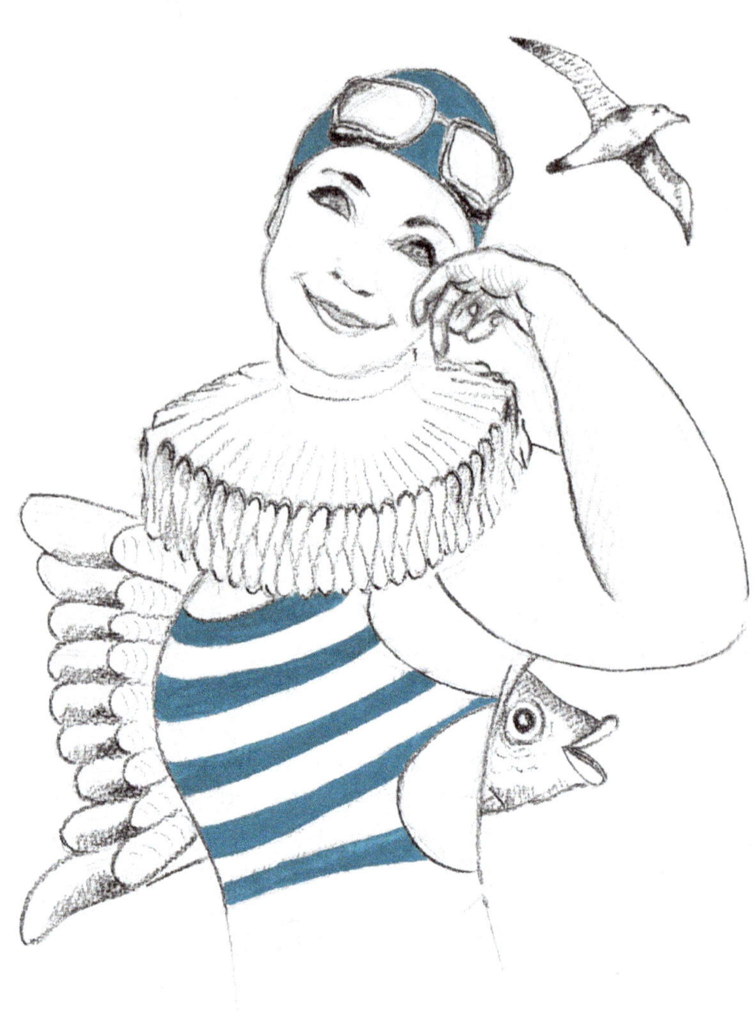

12. Further Embracing the Cold

As we've seen, sea bathing offers a wealth of benefits. What's more, taking winter dips in cold water often intensifies these advantages and introduces new ones. Multiple recent scientific studies confirm that regular cold-water immersion has a range of positive effects on health.

Let's greet the cold warmly!

Through a natural process called hormesis, when our body is exposed to a mild or short-term stressor, it generates a positive defensive and adaptive reaction, strengthening itself and developing greater resilience.

Cold water immersion acts as a stressor for the body. When practiced gradually and sensibly (following the rule of 1 minute per 1°C), our body adapts to the cold sensation over time. This practice naturally and progressively improves our body's strength, endurance, and capabilities.

Cold water bathing triggers the production of so-called survival and pleasure hormones: adrenaline, dopamine, and serotonin. This results in a profound euphoric feeling of happiness that can last from 12 to 72 hours, along with reduced anxiety.
As a result, our bodies learn to handle daily stress more calmly.

Our mental resilience is put to the test, with positive effects on our willpower, mindset, energy levels, and ability to concentrate.

Regular cold water baths stimulate and enhance our immune system's activity, making it more effective through hormonal production and a chain of defense reactions.

Our metabolism increases, our ability to adapt to daily temperature drops and our thermogenesis strengthen, and weight regulation improves effortlessly.

Cold or even icy water, already widely used in sports, reduces inflammation and pain while promoting muscle recovery.

Our sleep also benefits from this practice, which has a calming and relaxing effect.

A study on insects, worms, and fish exposed to colder environments showed a significant increase in life expectancy for all these animals!

A certain addiction can develop with sea bathing, leading to frustration when the practice is not possible. Occasionally, we can partially fill this void with cold showers.

From each bath, we emerge stronger!

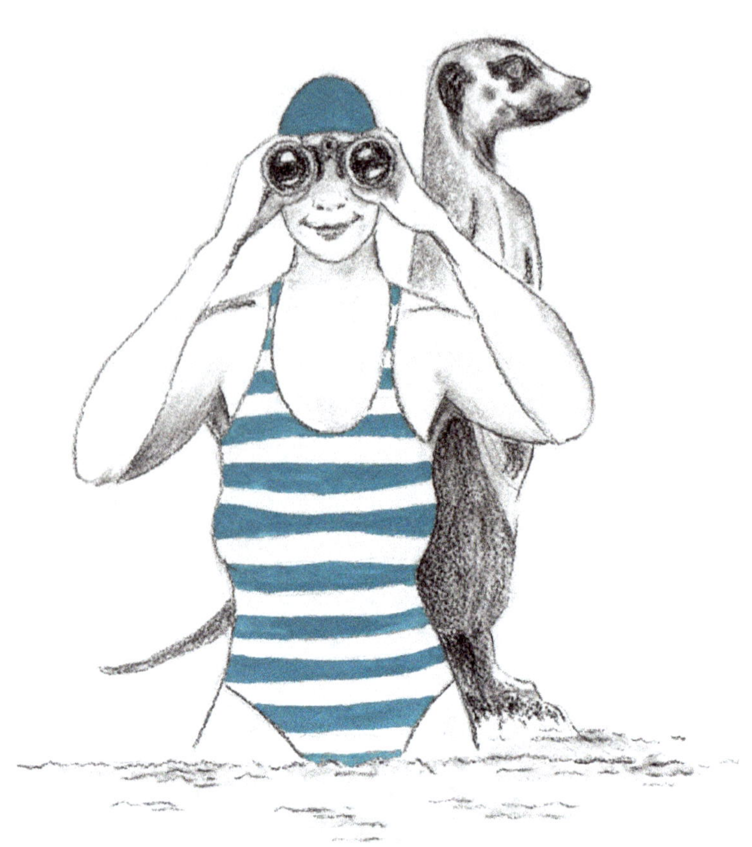

13. Socializing for Our Health

Some swimming clubs, groups, and rowing circles have existed for a very long time. To name just a few: the Brighton Swimming Club since 1860, London's Serpentine Swimming Club (river swimming) since 1864, and the Dolphin Club in San Francisco since 1877.
These institutions have long understood the virtues of shared experiences.
They cultivate camaraderie around their members' shared passion as both an art and a philosophy.

Today, we're witnessing a revival of winter sea bathing and a return to this practice within dynamic groups, although it remains somewhat niche.

Taking a dip in the sea can be incredibly rewarding.
However, especially during winter, it does require a bit of willpower, motivation, personal preparation, some basic logistics, and safety considerations.
For all these reasons, it's often ideal and recommended to swim with others.
This allows us to share advice, express doubts, show enthusiasm, offer encouragement, extend dinner invitations, and create a wonderful sense of camaraderie within the group.

The social bonds that form from regular group sea swimming are particularly strong and rewarding. Just chatting with a few active members is enough to see this. Within this shared passion, numerous interactions develop: sensations, emotions, joys, new connections, and incredibly fulfilling exchanges.

Often, these shared experiences extend beyond the swim itself, continuing over a hot drink, a snack, or a meal, fostering deep discussions and strong friendships.

This social connection is a vital and well-recognized factor in promoting good health and longevity.

Every swim is an experience we want to share!

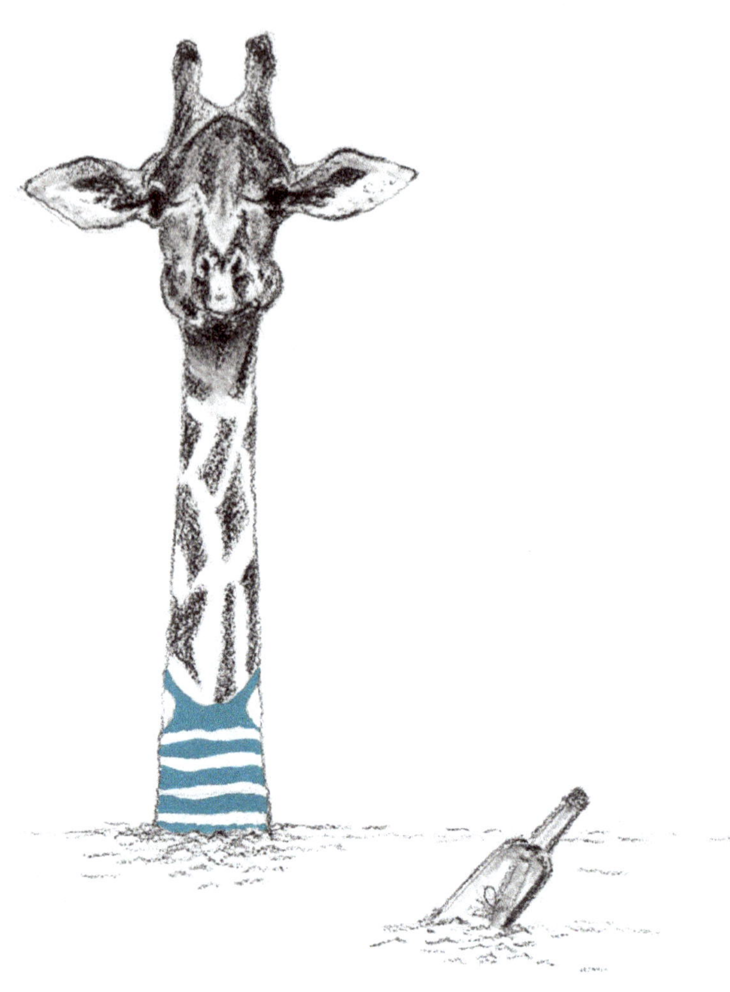

14. Blue Health, Blue Zones, Blue Therapies!

The color blue is universally associated with positive emotions: calm, serenity, credibility, wisdom, depth, openness, creativity, joy...
Attributed to Wallace J. Nichols

Bees are almost entirely insensitive to the color spectrum, with the notable exception of blue light.

Numerous international and multidisciplinary research programs—spanning fields such as immunology, biology, medicine, geography, health, sports, and psychology—are studying and measuring the remarkable therapeutic benefits of blue spaces. These areas, which include coastal regions, lakes, and rivers (even within urban settings), have been shown to positively impact our health, zest for life, optimism, and our relationships with others and the present moment.

The findings are striking and unanimous, prompting serious reflection on environmental design, architecture, and urban planning.

Surf therapy—referring to surf in its original sense, the foam formed by waves breaking on a seashore—is a pioneering blue health discipline. It advocates for various coastal activities, including swimming, bathing, walking, sailing, surfing, kayaking, rowing, and stand-up paddle-boarding.

The goal is to encourage these water-based practices or simply spending time by the sea, where the air is rich in minerals, trace elements, and negative ions.

This natural, preventive approach combats stress, depression, mental disorders, diabetes, cardiovascular diseases, obesity, addictions, sedentary lifestyles, and even post-traumatic stress disorders.

The benefits are numerous and inexpensive for those living near the coast.

Each swim extends our lifespan!

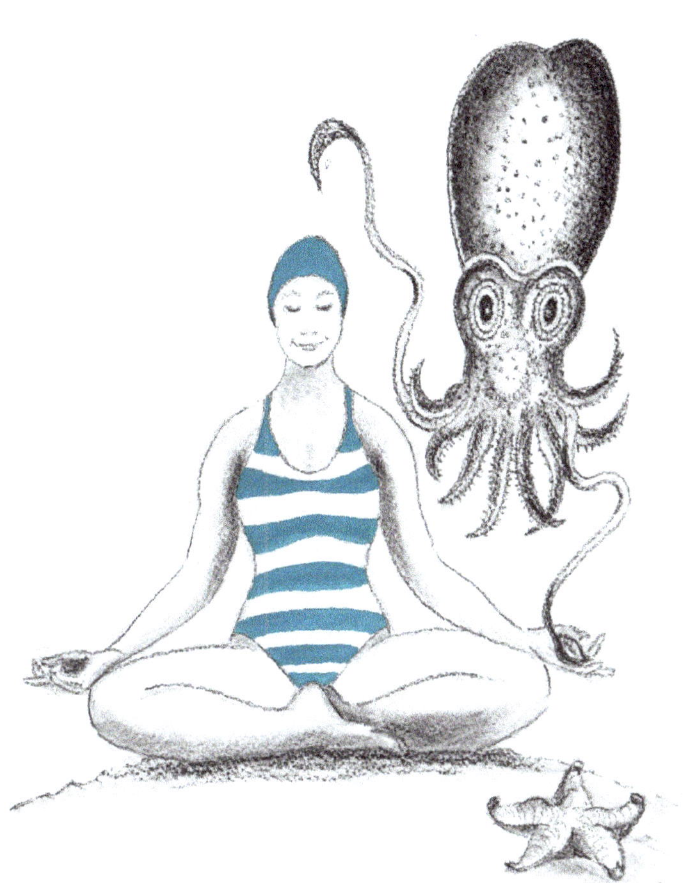

15. Caring for our beaches, seas, oceans, and planet

The ocean covers 70% of Earth's surface and stands as one of our most valuable resources. It's home to an immense biodiversity that feeds us, hydrates us, heals us, and contributes to our overall well-being.

The sea regulates our climate and weather patterns, playing a crucial role in maintaining our planet's balance and, by extension, our very existence.
However, this fragile ecosystem is under threat from industrial overfishing (which goes hand in hand with intensive agriculture and deforestation), offshore fossil fuel extraction, industrial and chemical pollution, plastic waste, and our often irresponsible behavior.

It is our duty to respect and protect our oceans with humility, humanity, and wisdom in order to preserve this extraordinary natural resource that sustains us, nourishes us, heals us, and on which we depend.

Practical tips for responsible swimmers and citizens, keeping in mind that ocean conservation starts with each of us!

Let's be mindful of our water usage.

Let's keep our seas clean by not throwing anything into the sea—trash, cigarette butts, oils, etc.

When it comes to seafood, let's make informed choices. Consider factors like species sustainability, origin, size, and fishing or farming methods.

Let's prioritize locally sourced products.

Let's reduce our carbon footprint by walking or cycling when possible, carpooling or using public transport, cutting down on energy consumption, and opting for green energy sources.

Let's avoid plastic—packaging, bottles—whenever possible; sort and recycle.

Let's compost our organic waste.

When needed, opt for sunscreens and oils that are gentle on both our skin and the oceans.

On the beach, embrace the natural tideline—those seaweeds and natural debris left by the tide. Mechanical cleaning destroys this valuable ecosystem. If cleaning is necessary, more eco-friendly methods exist.

Beach showers are a luxury that can lead to water waste. Let's use them mindfully.
Digital pollution is a rapidly growing environmental concern. Stay informed, be vigilant, and practice digital minimalism. Regulate our online habits and recycle our electronics.
Let's experience the sea with our own eyes rather than through our smartphones.

Our role is clear: to discover, love, understand, respect, protect, and remain committed to our oceans.

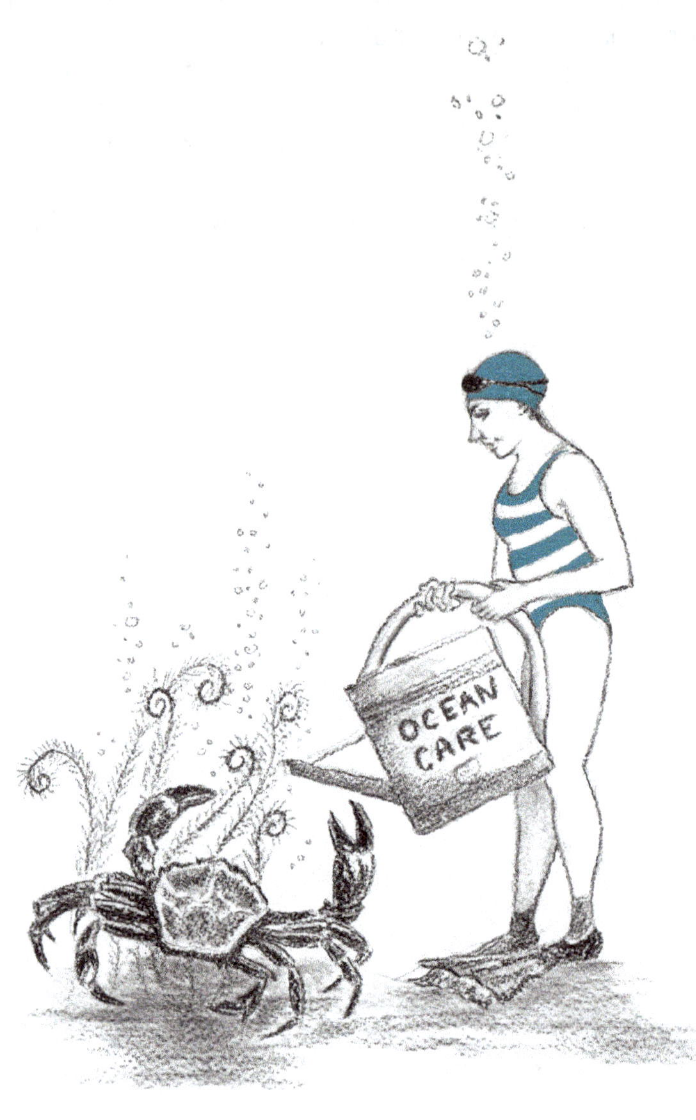
OCEAN
CARE

16. Practical Tips on How to Enjoy Sea Bathing

If it's been a while since your last check-up, or if you have any health concerns, ongoing treatments, heart problems, or blood pressure issues, consider getting a quick medical assessment for peace of mind.

Always check the weather forecast, tides, currents, baïnes, presence of jellyfish or weever fish, water quality, dangerous rocks, sharp shells, and be aware of boat traffic and navigation channels.

This guide is for everyone, from newborns to centenarians and beyond.

Preferably, sea bathing is done in swimwear for the best experience and maximum benefits.

Splash around, swim, and move your body at your own pace—this healthy activity has very few risks or contraindications

Nevertheless, here are some tips and precautions to keep in mind before diving in:
Avoid alcohol before bathing to stay alert, and preferably swim on an empty stomach. It's advisable to swim with a friend, especially when starting out in cool water.

Begin in summer or autumn, when the water temperature drops gradually.

Enter the water calmly, thoroughly wetting your hands, face, neck, and chest before fully immersing yourself.

Breathe slowly to find your rhythm and stay relaxed. The initial cool or cold sensation—which lasts about two minutes—will quickly subside during your swim and lessen with practice.

The duration of your swim is personal, depending on how you feel, your habits, and your current fitness level. There's no need for competition or record-breaking.

We all react differently to cold. A commonly cited rule suggests a maximum duration in minutes equal to the water temperature in Celsius.
For example, if the water is 15°C (59°F), aim for a maximum swim of 15 minutes.

Swimming parallel to the shore, where you can stand, is safe and ideal.
For swimming further out, it's highly recommended to use a swim buoy.

A buoy makes you visible from afar and provides a rest spot if you get tired or develop a cramp.

Consider wearing a swim cap and earplugs if you're swimming with your head underwater. This helps reduce the cold sensation, minimizes heat loss, and protects against ear infections and surfer's ear (also known as exostosis, a condition that can lead to hearing impairment).

Depending on the season, bring warm clothes suitable for the duration of your swim and perhaps a hot, post-swim beverage.

(NB Even in summer, we can never feel too hot after a cold swim.)

17. What to know about swimming in cool, cold (below 50°F/10°C), or even icy (below 41°F/5°C) water

Let's not forget that this activity should remain enjoyable!

Practice with others and gradually acclimate to colder water temperatures.
Learn to recognize your body's reactions and limits, and respect them.

Often, right after a winter swim, while still in our swimsuits, we don't feel the cold even as onlookers bundled in parkas and beanies watch us. We're overwhelmed by a sense of joy and fulfillment, riding a hormonal high. This special moment, known as the honeymoon phase, lasts only a few minutes. Make the most of it by drying off, putting on a warm wool hat, and bundling up. Remember, we lose about 30% of our body heat through our heads.

After getting out of the water, our body temperature continues to drop due to a phenomenon called afterdrop, which is caused by vasodilation. It's perfectly normal to experience shivers and shakes even after you've gotten dressed. This is simply a muscular reflex, like chills, that helps your body warm up.
Don't rush to take a hot shower right away. Instead, grab a snack in a warm place and let your body temperature rise naturally. This process can take anywhere from 30 minutes to an hour.

Taking a walk is also a great way to kickstart the warming process. However, it's best to avoid any intense physical activity after a winter swim.

Keep in mind that a cold swim starts at immersion and ends when your body returns to its normal temperature of about 98.6°F (37°C). It's crucial to consider this post-swim phase.

Staying in too long could reverse the desired effects, tire the body, and lead to hypothermia.

When sea bathing, it's important to take a gradual approach and listen to your body both during and after your time in the water. Start with short dips and moderate activity to get a feel for the sensations, then slowly increase your time and intensity at your own pace.

Remember to stay well-hydrated before and after your swim. Proper hydration is crucial for your body's ability to warm up effectively.

After each cold-water swim, we emerge feeling rejuvenated!

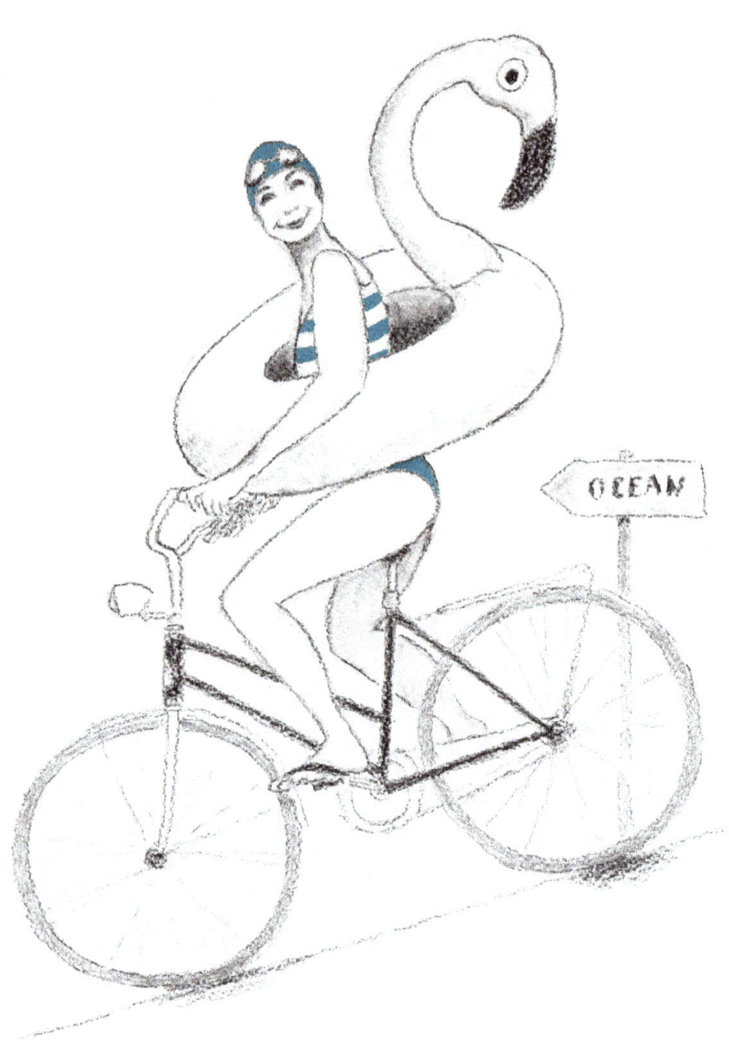

OCEAN

18. Cultivating Informed and responsible swimming habits

When venturing into new, unfamiliar, or different waters, approach with humility and curiosity. Always gather information before diving in.
Make it a habit to carry a mobile phone and remember to inform your loved ones about your swimming plans and location.

Jellyfish Stings

While generally harmless, be aware that tropical jellyfish stings can cause more intense symptoms, including discomfort, headaches, weakness, cramps...
If stung:
Calmly exit the water. Rinse thoroughly with seawater—never freshwater!
Apply fine sand to the affected area and gently scrape with a credit card or postcard. Rinse again with seawater and repeat if necessary.
If visible tentacle fragments remain in the skin, carefully remove them with tweezers.
For severe stings, the venom can be neutralized with vinegar.

Jellyfish venom is thermolabile, which means it can be destroyed by heat. You can treat the wound by applying heat with a hairdryer or hot water bottle.

Weever Fish Stings

The weever is a small fish, about 6 inches long, with venomous dorsal spines. It buries itself in shallow sandy areas.
Stings, although painful, are not fatal and occur when stepping on the fish or digging in the sand with hands, and cause immediate intense pain and swelling. Weever venom is also heat-sensitive. If possible, immerse the affected limb in very hot water—around 113°F (45°C)—for 15 minutes, or carefully heat the area with a hairdryer. Afterward, disinfect the wound.
When entering the water, drag your feet flat on the sandy bottom to scare away weever fish. You can also wear water shoes or sandals with soles for protection.

Types of rip currents known in France as "baïnes"

These offshore currents, found on beaches with waves, can pull swimmers out to sea. At low tide, you may notice shallow pools or depressions in the sand, which pose little danger. At high tide, these areas might be recognizable as calmer zones where waves don't break, and the water may appear darker.

If caught in a rip current, try not to panic, don't attempt to swim against it, signal for help, and swim parallel to the shore towards an area with breaking waves. The current will weaken, allowing you to return to the beach.

Cold Water Shock (Hydrocution)

Cold water shock occurs when body temperature is much higher than water temperature. It can cause loss of consciousness and lead to drowning.
To prevent this, especially after prolonged sun exposure, intense exercise, or a heavy meal with alcohol, enter the water gradually. Wet your hands, neck, face, chest, and arms. Pay attention to your body's reactions.
Swim with a friend for mutual supervision.
Symptoms include dizziness, vision problems, anxiety, extreme fatigue, feeling of ice-cold water, cramps, and headaches.

Hypothermia

This occurs when the body can't maintain its core temperature of 98.6°F (37°C). Mild hypothermia (97.7°F to 95°F / 36.5°C to 35°C) is common after winter swimming.

Symptoms include shivering, cold skin, and paleness.
Actions to take include covering up well, moving gently, going to a warm place, drinking a hot beverage, letting body temperature rise naturally, and taking a lukewarm shower, gradually increasing the temperature.

Severe hypothermia (95°F to 86°F / 35°C to 30°C) requires immediate attention. Symptoms include mottled skin, a strange gaze, dilated pupils, lack of coordination, and mental confusion.
Immediately seek emergency medical care if severe hypothermia is suspected.

When waiting for medical services:

Move the person to a warmer place if possible. Unless they are unconscious, keep them seated rather than lying down.
Once in a warmer location, remove any wet clothing.
Wrap the individual in a survival blanket, towels, or any warm clothing and/or protection, including a hat.
Offer a warm drink (no alcohol) and energy-rich foods (chocolate, sugar, etc.), but only if the person is able to eat and drink.
Monitor the individual's body temperature to ensure it increases and maintains an adequate level.

In cases of hypothermia, avoid certain actions:
Do not give a hot bath to a person with hypothermia.
Do not massage their limbs and body.
Do not give them alcohol to drink.

These actions can cause excessive and rapid vasodilation of blood vessels in the limbs. This can lead to a significant drop in blood pressure, potentially impacting the function of vital organs like the brain, heart, lungs, and kidneys.

We're ready to fully enjoy the ocean—let's be its ambassador!

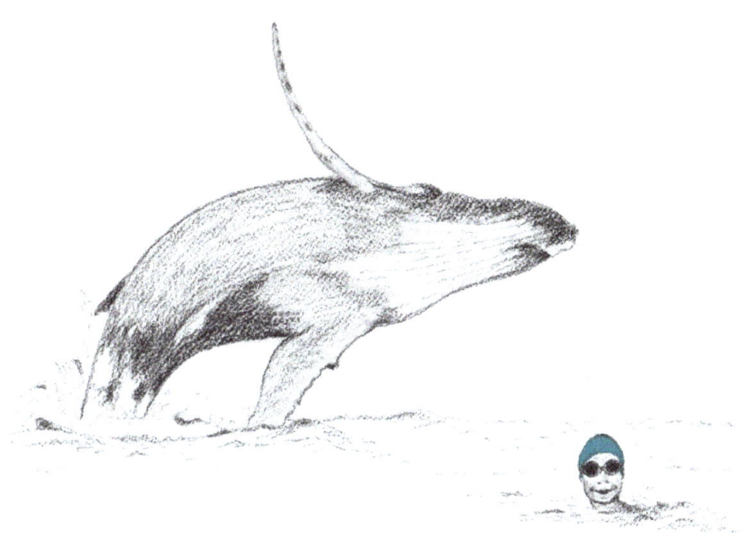

19. Bibliography

Detoxseafication, Dr Guillaume Barucq,
Surf Prevention edition

Surf thérapie, Dr Guillaume Barucq,
Surf Prevention edition

La santé bleue, Pascale d'Erm, Masson edition

Swimming to Antarctica, Lynne Cox, Knopf edition

Open Water Swimming Manual, Lynne Cox,
Knopf edition

Blue Mind, Wallace J. Nichols, Abacus edition

Journal de Nage, Chantal Thomas

Toumo training, cold yoga performed with Maurice Daubard.

Wim Hof cold and breathing training performed with Jean François Tual.

Meetings or exchanges with extreme swimmers such as Jaimie Monahan, Jacques Tuset, Doctor Alexandre Fuzeau.

S.N.S.M website
Société Nationale de Sauvetage en Mer

Website: OUTDOORSWIMMER.COM

Article from Department of Applied Physiology and Kinesiology of Florida: Research on effect of cold water temperature.

Personal experiences: professional diver and regular winter swimmer in cold and icy waters.

www.ingramcontent.com/pod-product-compliance
Lightning Source LLC
Chambersburg PA
CBHW050826250726
48653CB00006B/2451